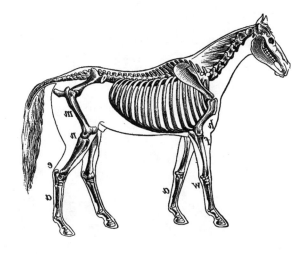

The Horse Anatomy

Coloring Book

For Equestrians

The earliest any horse is fully physically developed is 5.5 to 6.5 years of age. And that's the minimum. Many horses mature after this. Our first role as a horse owner is to do no damage to the horse's long term health, and not ask too much of them too young

Elaine Heney

14x _____

13x _____

13 _____

14 _____

16 _____

11 _____

15 _____

15x _____

9 _____

12 _____

19 _____

21 _____

20 _____

27 _____

22 _____

26 _____

23 _____

29 _____

24 _____

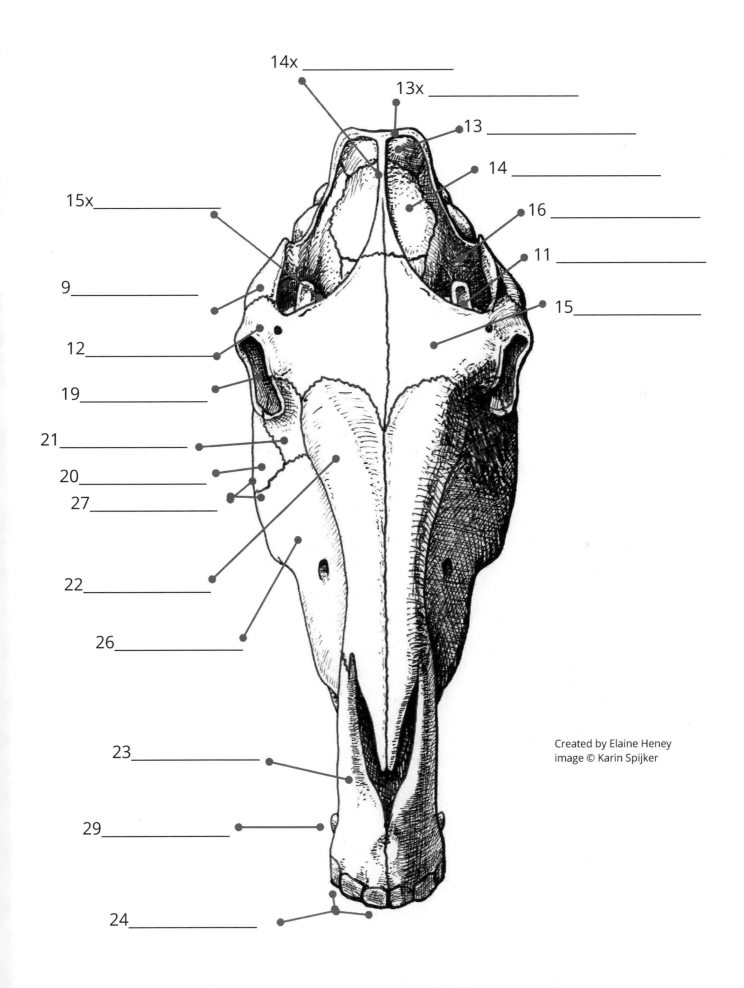

Created by Elaine Heney
image © Karin Spijker

Answers:

9: Arcus zycomaticus

11: Proc. coronoideus of the lower jawbone

12: Orbital arch

13: Os occipitale

13x: Crest of os occipitale

14: Os Parietale

14x: Crest of the os parietale

15: Os frontale

15x: Frontal crests

16: Os temporale

19: Orbita

20: Os jugale

21: Os lacrimale

22: Os nasale

23: Os intermaxillare s. incisivum

24: Upper incisor teeth

26: os maxillare sup.

27: Zygomatic or facial crest

29: Lower canine tooth, exposed from the alveolus

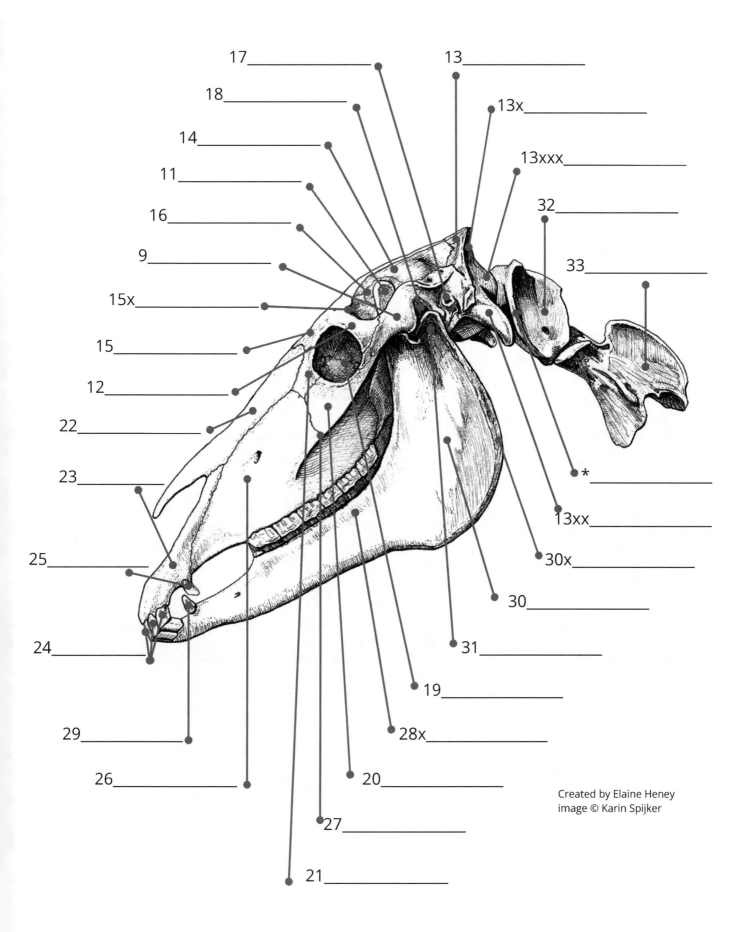

17_____

13_____

18_____

13x_____

14_____

13xxx_____

11_____

32_____

16_____

9_____

33_____

15x_____

15_____

12_____

22_____

*_____

23_____

13xx_____

25_____

30x_____

24_____

30_____

31_____

29_____

19_____

26_____

28x_____

27_____

20_____

21_____

Created by Elaine Heney
image © Karin Spijker

Answers:

11: Proc. coronoideus of the lower jawbone

16: Os temporale

9: Arcus zycomaticus

15x: Frontal crest

15: Os frontale

12: Orbital arch

22: Os nasale

23: OS intermaxillare s. incisivum

25: Upper canine tooth

24: upper incisor teeth

29: Lower canine tooth, exposed from alveolus

26: Os maxillare sup.

21: Os lacrimale

27: Zygomatic or facial crest

20: Os jugale

28x: Body of the lower jawbone

19: Orbita

31: Condyle process of the lower jaw

30: Branch of the lower jaw

30x: Angle of the lower jaw

13xx: Jugular process of os occipitale

*: Ala border of atlas

13: Os occipitale

13x: Crest of os occipitale

13xxx: Condyle of the os occipitale

32: 1st cervical vertebra (Atlas)

33: 2nd cervical vertebra

14: Os parietale

17: Meatus acusticus externus

18: Temporo-maxilliary joint

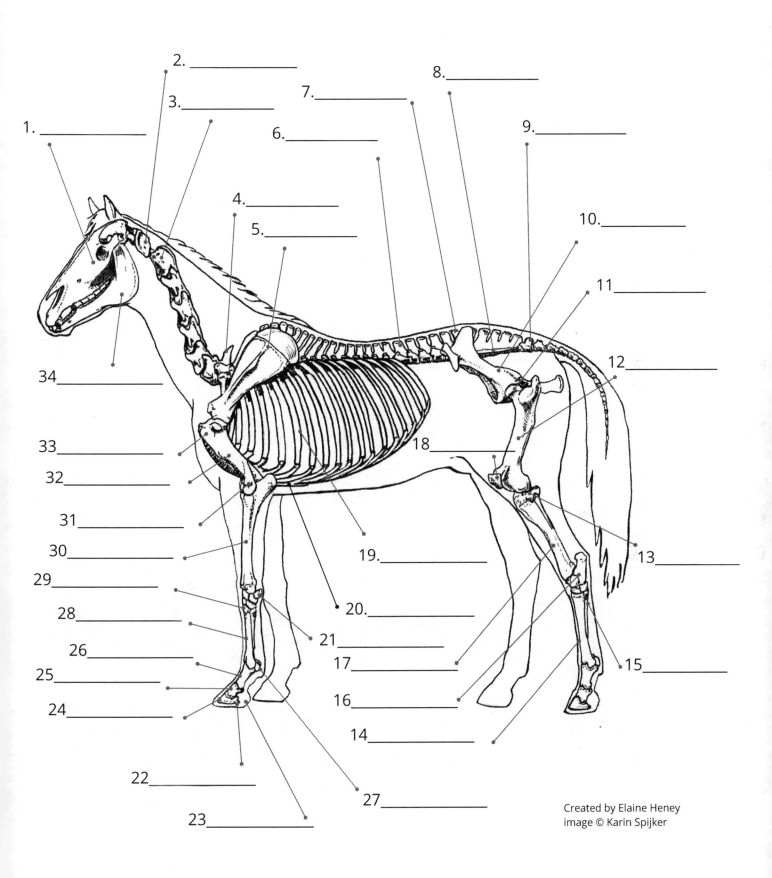

1. _____

2. _____

3. _____

4. _____

5. _____

6. _____

7. _____

8. _____

9. _____

10. _____

11. _____

12. _____

13. _____

14. _____

15. _____

16. _____

17. _____

18. _____

19. _____

20. _____

21. _____

22. _____

23. _____

24. _____

25. _____

26. _____

27. _____

28. _____

29. _____

30. _____

31. _____

32. _____

33. _____

34. _____

Answers:

1. Skull
2. Atlas
3. Axis
4. First thoracic vertebra
5. Shoulder blade
6. First lumbar vertebra
7. Point of hip
8. Lumbosacral joint
9. First tail vertebra
10. Pelvis
11. Hip joint
12. Femur
13. Stifle joint
14. Cannon bone
15. Splint bone
16. Hock
17. Tibia
18. Patella
19. Rib cage
20. Sternum
21. Pisiform bone
22. Navicular bone
23. Lateral cartlilage
24. Pedal bone
25. Short pastern bone
26. Long pastern bone
27. Sesamoid bone
28. Cannon bone
29. Knee
30. Radius
31. Elbow
32. Humerus
33. Point of shoulder
34. Jaw

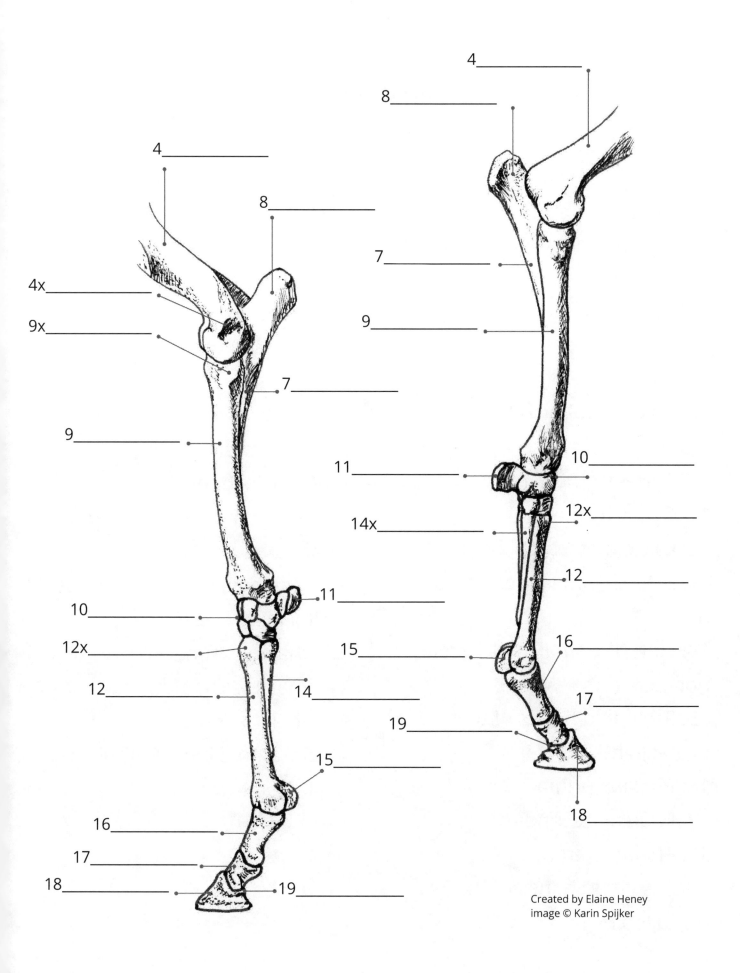

4_____

8_____

4x_____

9x_____

7_____

9_____

10_____

12x_____

12_____

14_____

15_____

16_____

17_____

18_____

19_____

4_____

8_____

7_____

9_____

11_____

14x_____

10_____

12x_____

12_____

15_____

16_____

17_____

19_____

18_____

11_____

Created by Elaine Heney
image © Karin Spijker

Answers:

4: Humerus

4x: External or extensor condyle of the humerus

7: Ulna

8: Olecranon

9: Radius

9x: External tuberosity of the radius

10: Bones of the carpus

11: Os pisiforme

12: Large metacarpal bone

14: External small metacarpal bone

14x: Internal small metacarpal bone

15: Sesamoid bones of the 1st digital joint

16: Phalanx prima

17: Phalanx secunda

18: Phalanx tertia

19: Sesamoid bones of the 3rd digital point

4: Humerus

7: Ulna

8: Olecranon

9: Radius

10: Bones of the carpus

11: Os pisiforme

12: Large metacarpal bone

12x: Tuberosity of large metacarpal bone

14x: Internal small metacarpal bone

15: Sesamoid bones of the 1st digital joint

16: Phalanx prima

17: Phalanx secunda

18: Phalanx tertia

19: Sesamoid bones of the 3rd digital joint

4_____

4x_____

9x_____

9_____

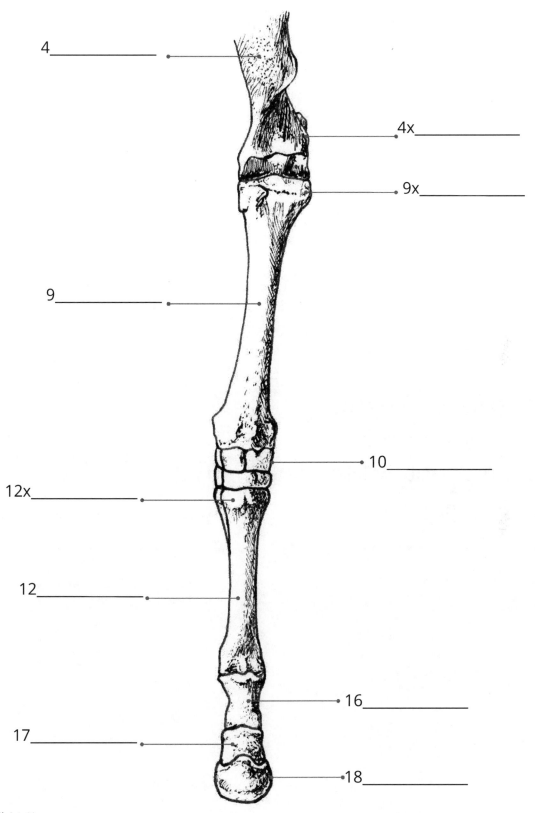

10_____

12x_____

12_____

16_____

17_____

18_____

Answers:

4: Humerus

4x: External or extensor condyle of the humerus

9: Radius

9x: External tuberosity of the radius

10: Bones of the carpus

12: Large metacarpal bone

12x: Tuberosity of large metacarpal bone

16: Phalanx prima

17: Phalanx secunda

18: Phalanx tertia

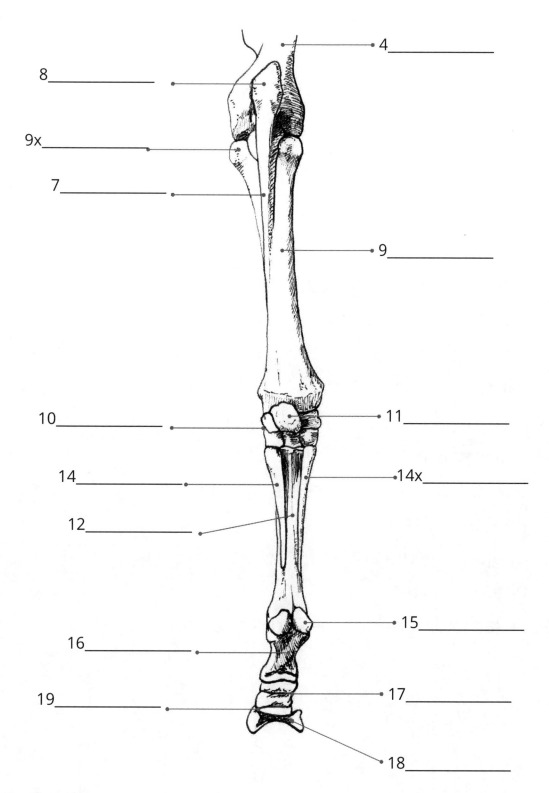

8 _____

9x _____

7 _____

4 _____

9 _____

10 _____

11 _____

14 _____

14x _____

12 _____

15 _____

16 _____

19 _____

17 _____

18 _____

Answers:

4: Humerus

7:Ulna

8: Olecranon

9: Radius

9x: External tuberosity of the radius

10: Bones of the carpus

11: Os pisiforme

12: Large metacarpal bone

14: External small metacarpal bone

14x: Internal small metacarpal bone

15: Sesamoid bones of the 1st digital joint

16: Phalanx prima

17: Phalanx secunda

18: Phalanx tertia

19: Sesamoid bones of the 3rd digital joint

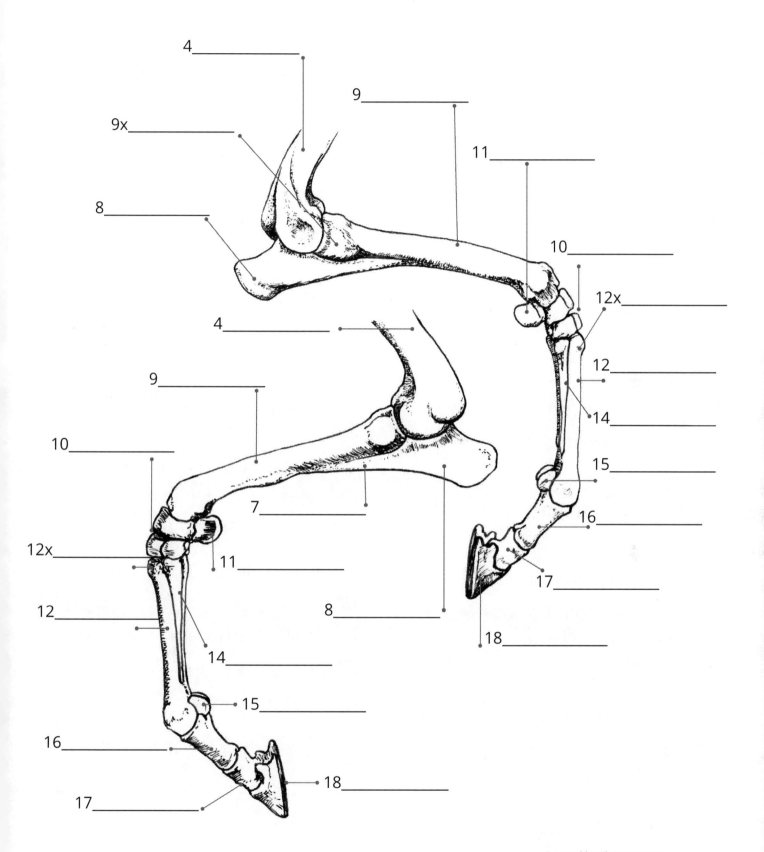

4 _____

9x_____

9 _____

8 _____

11 _____

10 _____

12x_____

12 _____

14 _____

15 _____

16 _____

17 _____

18 _____

4 _____

9 _____

10 _____

7 _____

11 _____

12x_____

12 _____

14 _____

15 _____

16 _____

17 _____

18 _____

8 _____

Answers:

4: Humerus

8: Olecranon

9: Radius

9x: External tuberosity of the radius

10: Bones of the carpus

11: Os pisiforme

12: Large metacarpal bone

12x: Tuberosity of large metacarpal bone

14: External small metacarpal bone

15: Sesamoid bones of the 1st digital joint

16: Phalanx prima

17: Phalanx secunda

18: Phalanx tertia

4: Humerus

7: Ulna

8: Olecranon

9: Radius

10: Bones of the carpus

11: Os pisiforme

12: Large metacarpal bone

12x: Tuberosity of large metacarpal bone

14: External small metacarpal bone

15: Sesamoid bones of the 1st digital joint

16: Phalanx prima

17: Phalanx secunda

18: Phalanx tertia

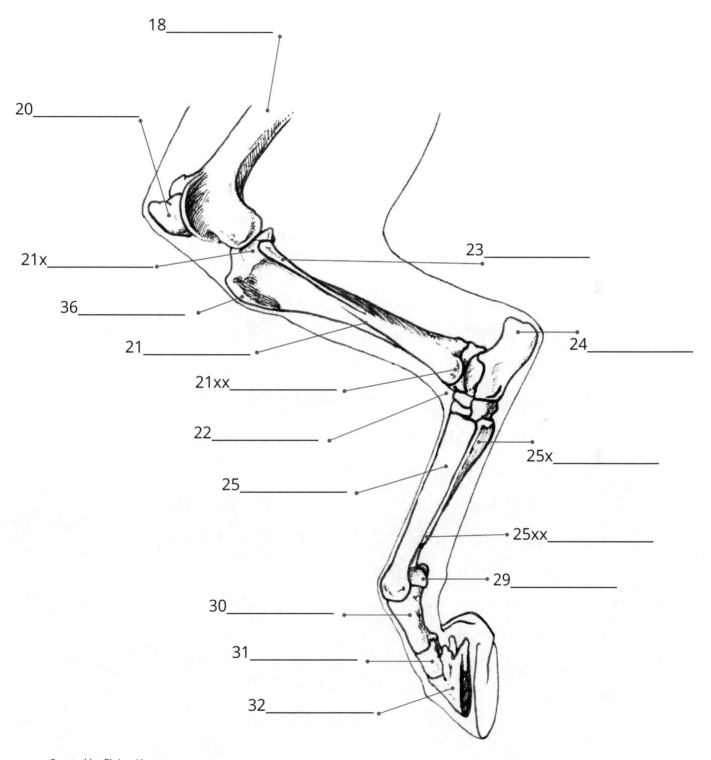

18_____

20_____

21x_____

36_____

21_____

21xx_____

22_____

25_____

23_____

24_____

25x_____

25xx_____

29_____

30_____

31_____

32_____

Answers:

18: Lower end of femur

20: Patella

21: Tibia

21x: External condyle of tibia

21xx: External malleolus of tibia

22: Tarsus

23: Fibula

24: Tuber calcanei

25: Large metatarsal bone

25x: Inner small metatarsal bone

25xx: Nodular enlarged end of the inner small metatarsal bone

29: Sesamoid bone of the 1st digital joint

30: Phalanx prima

31: Phalanx secunda

32: Phalanx tertia

36: Crista tibiae

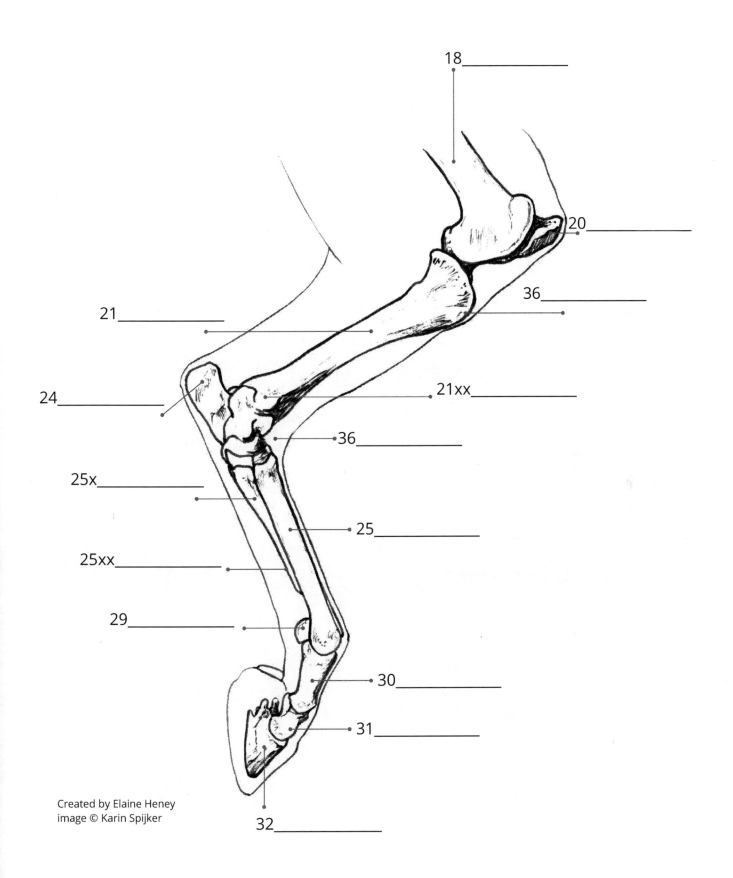

18_____

20_____

36_____

21_____

24_____

21xx_____

36_____

25x_____

25_____

25xx_____

29_____

30_____

31_____

32_____

Created by Elaine Heney
image © Karin Spijker

Answers:

18: Lower end of femur

20: Patella

21: Tibia

21x: External condyle of tibia

21xx: External malleolus of tibia

24: Tuber calcanei

25: Large metatarsal bone

25x: Inner small metatarsal bone

25xx: Nodular enlarged end of the inner small metatarsal bone

29: Sesamoid bone of the 1st digital point

30: Phalanx prima

31: Phalanx secunda

32: Phalanx tertia

36: Crista tibiae

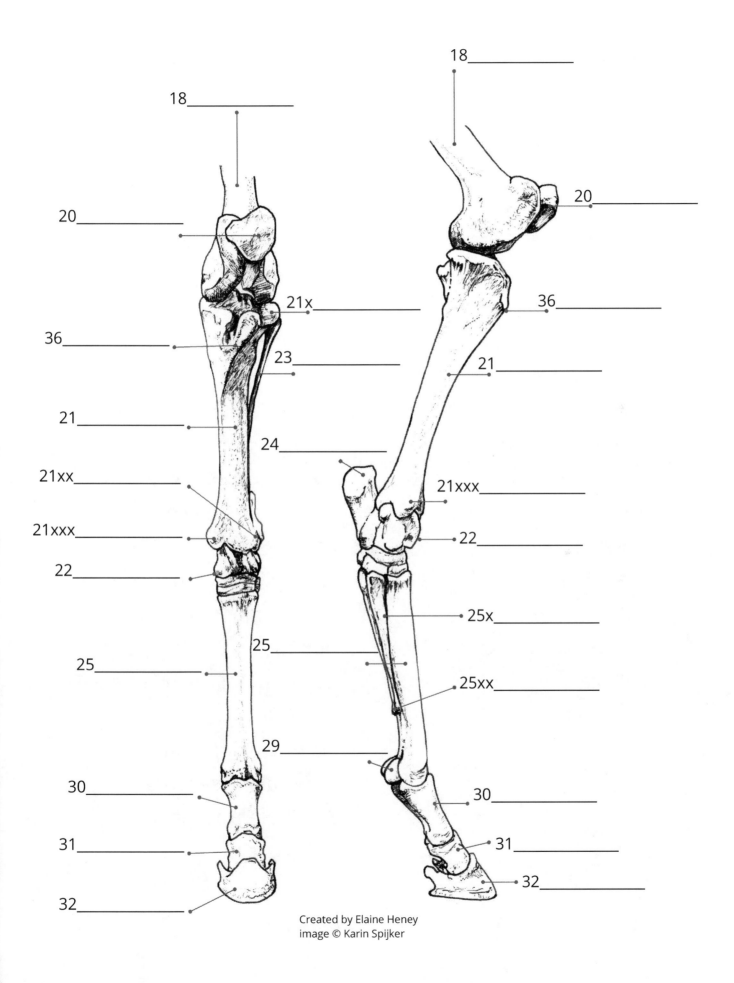

18_____

18_____

20_____

20_____

21x_____

36_____

36_____

23_____

21_____

21_____

24_____

21xx_____

21xxx_____

21xxx_____

22_____

22_____

25x_____

25_____

25_____

25xx_____

29_____

30_____

30_____

31_____

31_____

32_____

32_____

Created by Elaine Heney
image © Karin Spijker

Answers:

18: Lower end of femur

20: Patella

21: Tibia

21x: External condyle of tibia

21xx: External malleolus of tibia

21xxx: Internal malleolus of tibia

22: Tarsus

23: Fibula

25: Large metatarsal bone

30: Phalanx prima

31: Phalanx secunda

32: Phalanx tertia

36: Crista tibiae

18: Lower end of femur

20: Patella

21: Tibia

21xxx: Internal malleolus of tibia

22: Tarsus

24: Tuber calcanei

25: Large metatarsal bone

25x: Inner small metatarsal bone

25xx: Nodular enlarged end of the inner small metatarsal bone

29: Sesamoid bone of the 1st digital joint

30: Phalanx prima

31: Phalanx secunda

32: Phalanx tertia

36: Crista tibiae

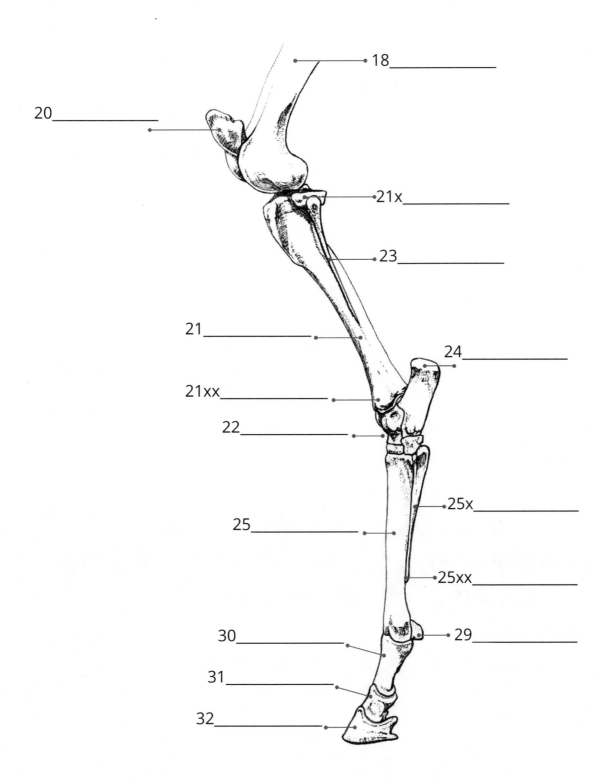

18_____

20_____

21x_____

23_____

21_____

24_____

21xx_____

22_____

25x_____

25_____

25xx_____

30_____

29_____

31_____

32_____

Answers:

18: Lower end of femur

20: Patella

21: Tibia

21x: External condyle of tibia

21xx: External malleolus of tibia

22: Tarsus

23: Fibula

24: Tuber calcanei

25: Large metatarsal bone

25x: Inner small metatarsal bone

25xx: Nodular enlarged end of the inner small metatarsal bone

29: Sesamoid bone of the 1st digital joint

30: Phalanx prima

31: Phalanx secunda

32: Phalanx tertia

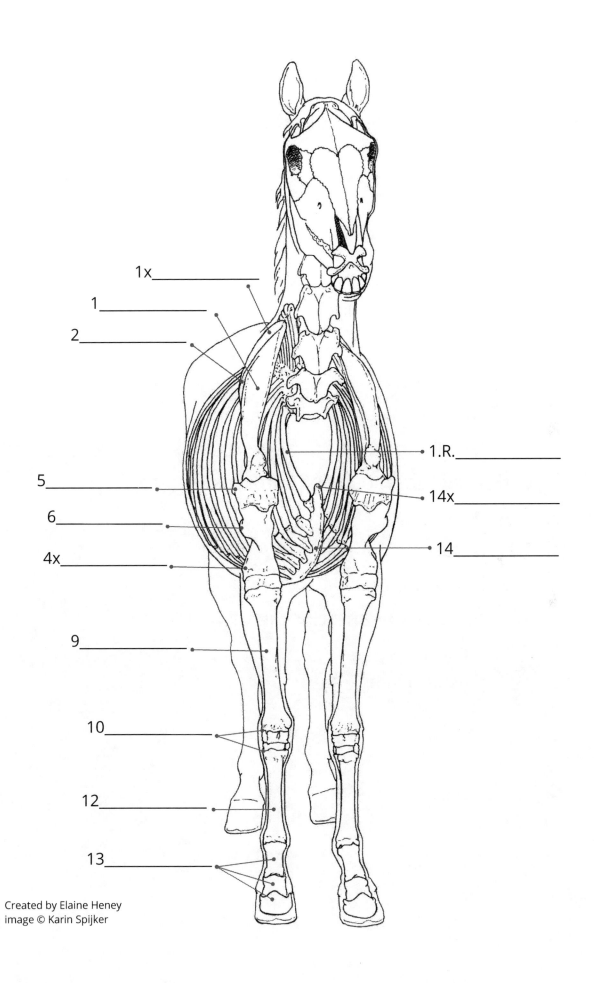

1x_____

1_____

2_____

1.R._____

5_____

14x_____

6_____

4x_____

14_____

9_____

10_____

12_____

13_____

Created by Elaine Heney
image © Karin Spijker

Answers:

1: Scapula

1x: Cartilago scapulae

1.R.: 1st Rib

2: Spina scapulae

4x: External epicondyle of humerus

5: External tuberosity of humerus

6: Deltoid tubersosity of humerus (rotator)

9: Radius

10: Carpus

12: Metacarpus

13: Phalanges of anterior digit

14: Sternum

14x: Cariniform cartilage

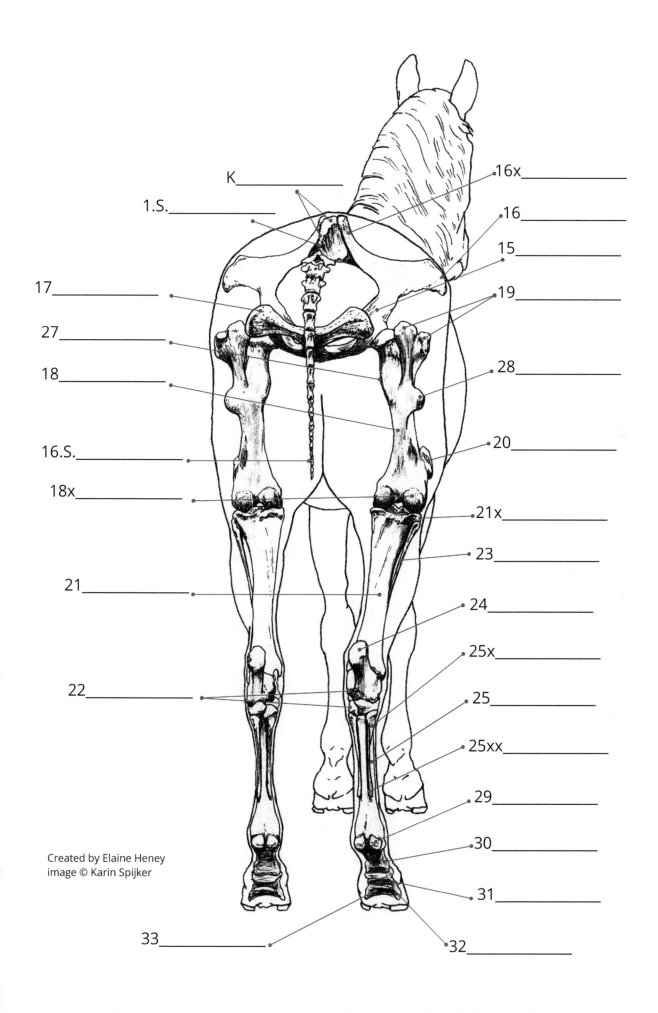

K_____

1.S._____

16x_____

16_____

15_____

17_____

19_____

27_____

18_____

28_____

16.S._____

20_____

18x_____

21x_____

23_____

21_____

24_____

25x_____

22_____

25_____

25xx_____

29_____

30_____

33_____

31_____

32_____

Created by Elaine Heney
image © Karin Spijker

Answers:

K: Sacrum

1.S.: 1st Caudal vertebra

15: Ossa pelvis

16: Tuber Coxae

16x: Tuber sacrale

16.S.: 16th caudal vertebra

17: Tuber ischii

18: Femur

18x: External condyle of the femur

19: Trochanter major of the femur

20: Patella

21: Tibia

21x: External condyle of the tibia

22: Tarsus

23: Fibula

24: Tuber calcanei

25: Large cannon bone (3rd metatarsal bone)

25x: External small cannon or splint bone (4th metatarsal bone)

25xx: Capitulum

27: Internal trochanter of the femur

28: External trochanter of the femur

29: Sesamoid bones of the 1st digital joint

30: Phalanx prima

31: Phalanx secunda

32: Phalanx tertia

33: Sesamoid bone of the 3rd digital point

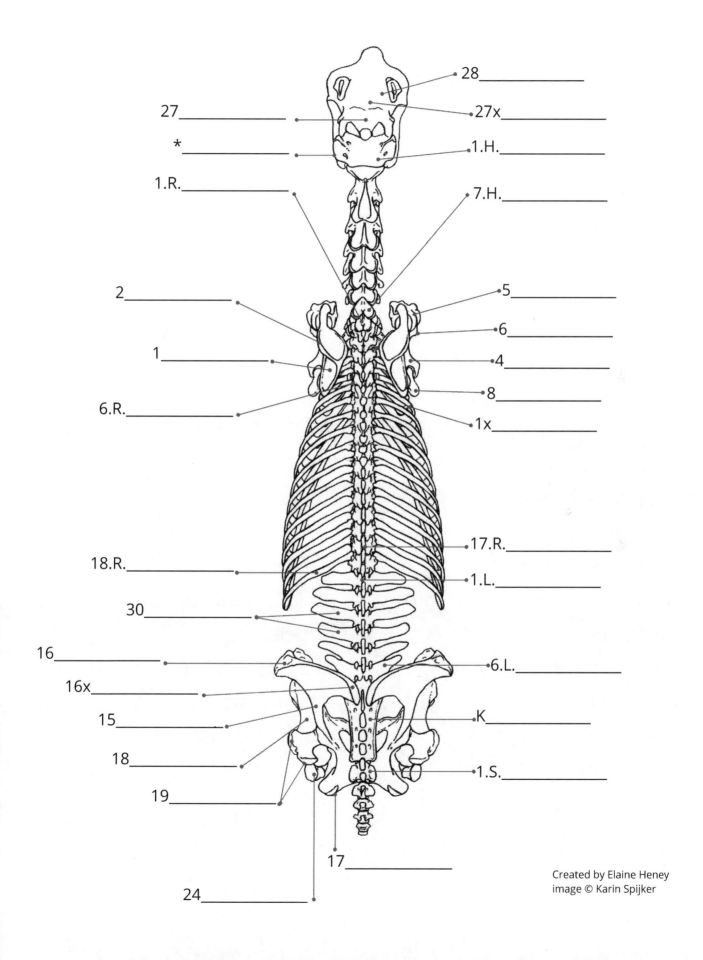

28_____

27_____   27x_____

*_____   1.H._____

1.R._____   7.H._____

2_____   5_____

1_____   6_____

6.R._____   4_____

8_____

1x_____

17.R._____

18.R._____   1.L._____

30_____

16_____   6.L._____

16x_____

15_____   K_____

18_____   1.S._____

19_____

17_____

24_____

Created by Elaine Heney
image © Karin Spijker

Answers:

*: Ala border of the atlas

K: Sacrum

1: Scapula

1x: Cartilago scapulae

1.H.: 1st cervical vertebra (atlas)

1.L.: 1st lumbar vertebra

1.R.: 1st thoraic (dorsal) vertebra

1.S.: 1st caudal vertebra

2: Spina scapulae

4: Humerus

5: External tuberosity

6: Deltoid tubersosity of the humerus

6.L.: 6th lumbar vertebra

6.R.: 6th rib

7.H.: 7th cervical vertebra

8: Olecranon

15: Pelvis

16: Tuber coxae

16x: Tuber sacrale

17: Tuber ischii

17.R.: 17 thoraic (dorsal) vertebra

18: Os femoris

18.R.: 18th rib

19: Trochanter major of the femur

24: Tuber calcanei

27: Os occipitale

27x: External occiptital tubersosity

28: Os parietale

30: Transverse processes of the lumbar vertebrae

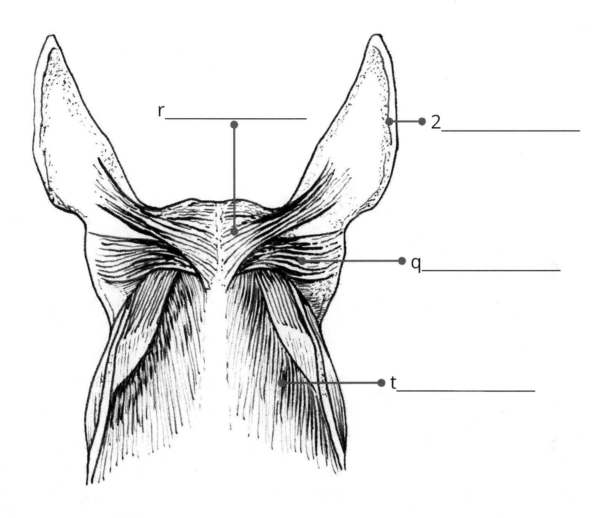

r_____

2_____

q_____

t_____

Answers:

r: Levator of the auricle

2: External or posterior edge of auricle

q: Abductor of the auricle

t: M. splenius

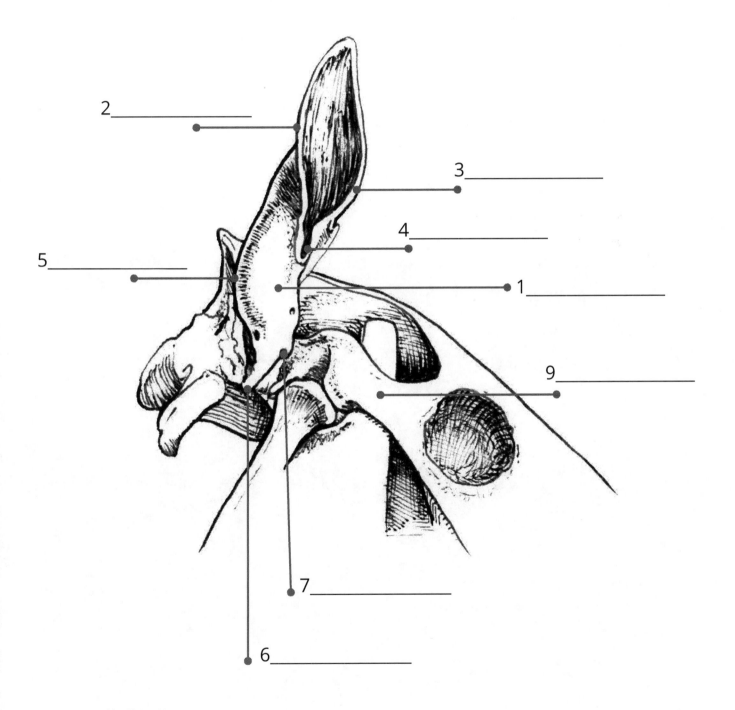

2_____

3_____

4_____

5_____

1_____

9_____

7_____

6_____

Answers:

1: Auricula or cartilage of the ear

2: External or posterior edge of auricle

3: Internal or anterior edge of auricle

4: Incisura intertragica

5: Base of auricle

6: Styloid process of auricle

7: Cartilago annularis

9: Arcus zycomaticus

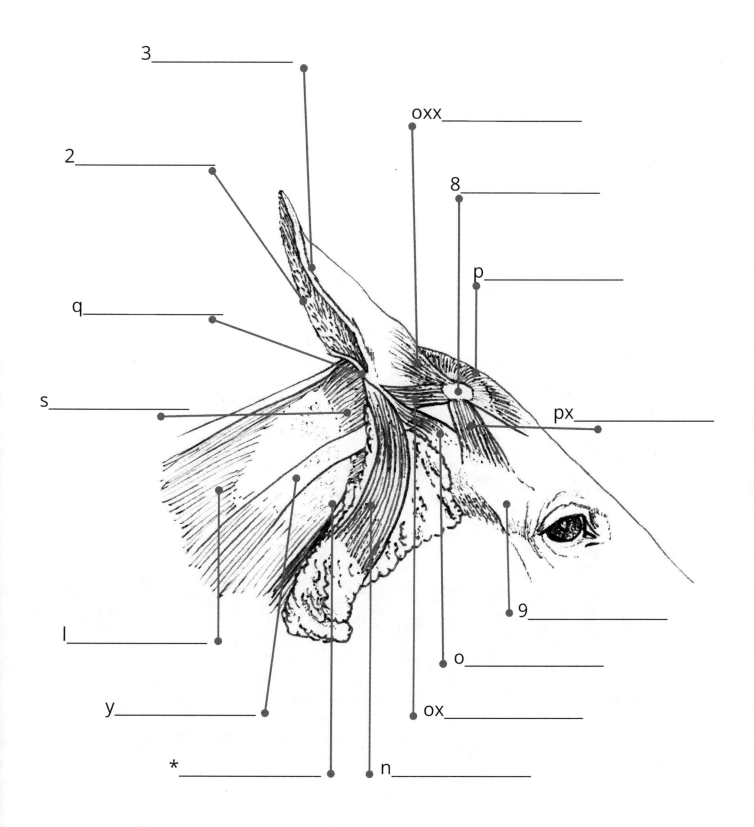

3_____

oxx_____

2_____

8_____

p_____

q_____

s_____

px_____

l_____

9_____

y_____

o_____

*_____

ox_____

n_____

Created by Elaine Heney
image © Karin Spijker

Answers:

*: Ala border of the atlas

2: External or posterior edge of auricle

3: Internal or posterior edge of auricle

8: Scutellum

9: Arcus annularis

l: M. dilatator nasi

n: Depressor of the auricle

o: External abductor of the auricle

ox: Inferior abductor of the auricle

oxx: Superior abductor of the auricle

p: M. scutularis

px: M. scutularis

s: M. obliquus capitis superior

q: Abductor of the auricle

y: Tendon of the M. longissimus capitis et atlantis

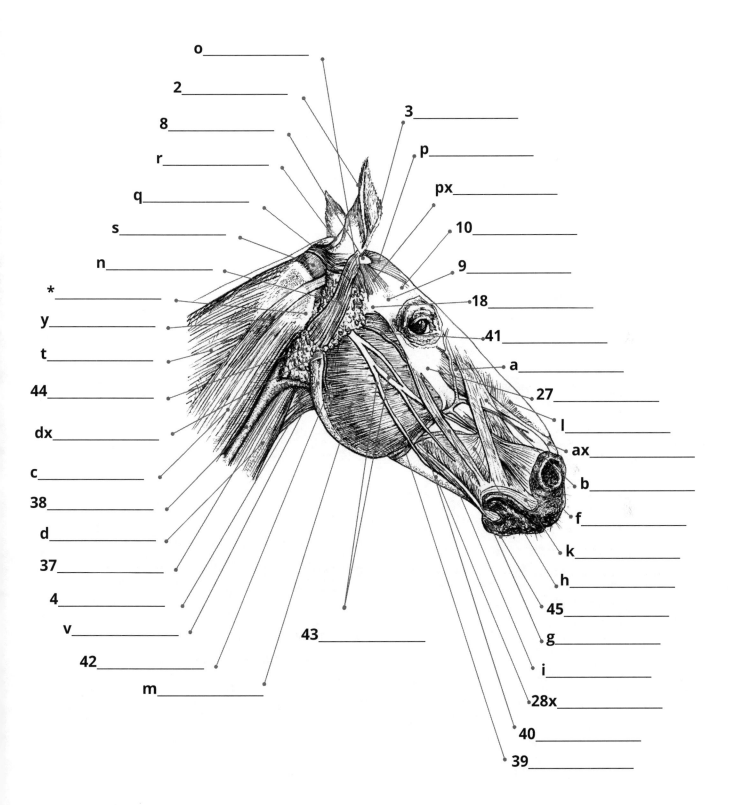

o_____

2_____

8_____

r_____

q_____

s_____

n_____

*_____

y_____

t_____

44_____

dx_____

c_____

38_____

d_____

37_____

4_____

v_____

42_____

m_____

3_____

p_____

px_____

10_____

9_____

18_____

41_____

a_____

27_____

l_____

ax_____

b_____

f_____

k_____

h_____

45_____

g_____

i_____

28x_____

40_____

39_____

43_____

Answers:

o: External adductor of the auricle

2: External or posterior edge of auricle

8: Scutellum

r:Levator of the auricle

q: Abductor of the auricle

s: M. obliquus capitis superior

n: Depressor of the auricle

*: Ala border of atlas

y: Tendon of the M. longissimus capitis

t: M. splenius

44: Glandula parotis

dx: Tendon at the end of M. sterno-mandibularis

c: Origin of the M. sterno-cleidomastoideus

38: V. jugularis

d: End of the M. sterno-mandibularis

37: V. maxillaris externa

4: Incisura intertragica

v: M. biventer maxillae, M. digastricus

42: Masseteric vein

m: M. masseter

43: Facial nerve

39: V. facialis

40: Ductus parotideus

28x: Body of the lower jawbone

i: M quadratus labii inferioris

g: M. zygomaticus major

45: Chin

h: M. buccinator

k: M. orbicularis oris

f: M. canisus s. pyramidalis nasi

b: M. levator labii sup. alaeque nasi

ax: Uniting tendon

l: M. dilatator nasi

27: Zygomatic or facial crest

a: M. levator labii sup propius

41: Transverse facial vein

18: Temporo-maxillary joint

9: Arcus zycomaticus

10: Temporal fossa

px: M. scutularis

p: M. scutularis

3: Internal or anterior edge of auricle

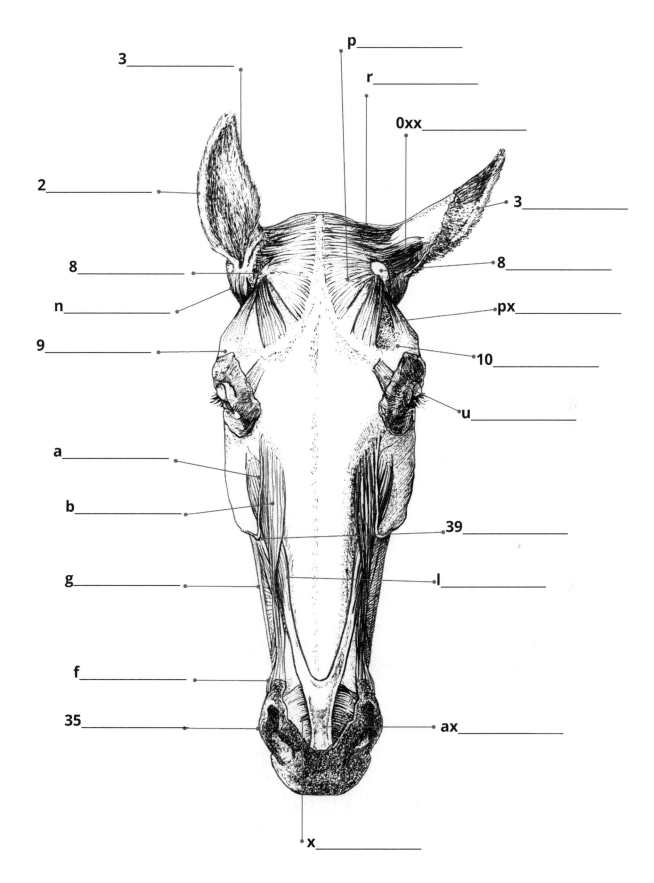

3_____

p_____

r_____

0xx_____

2_____

3_____

8_____

8_____

n_____

px_____

9_____

10_____

u_____

a_____

b_____

39_____

g_____

l_____

f_____

35_____

ax_____

x_____

Answers:

3: Internal or anterior edge of auricle

2: External or anterior edge of auricle

8: Scutellum

n: Depressor of the auricle

9: Arcus zycomaticus

a: M. levator labii sup. propius

b: M. levator labii sup. alaeque nasi

g: M. zygomaticus major

f: M. caninus s. pyramidalis nasi

35: The X shaped or alar cartilage of the nose

x: M. transversus nasi

ax: Uniting tendon

l: M. dilator nasi

39: V. facialis

u: M. corrugator supercilii

10: Temporal fossa

px: M. scutularis

8: Scutellum

3: Internal or anterior edge of auricle

oxx: Superior adductor of the auricle

r: Levator of the auricle

p: M. scutularis

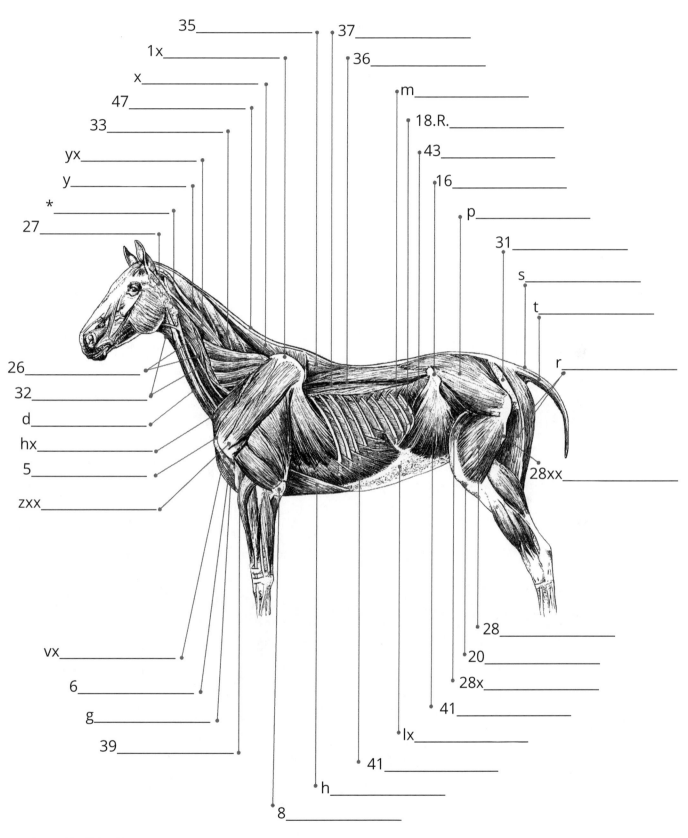

35_____
1x_____
x_____
47_____
33_____
yx_____
y_____
*_____
27_____

37_____
36_____
m_____
18.R._____
43_____
16_____
p_____
31_____
s_____
t_____
r_____

26_____
32_____
d_____
hx_____
5_____
zxx_____

28xx_____

vx_____
6_____
g_____
39_____

28_____
20_____
28x_____
41_____
lx_____
41_____
h_____
8_____

Answers:

26: Articular processes of the cervical vertebrae

32: M. omohyoideus

d: M. sternomandibularis

hx: Scapular portion of the M. pectoralis minor

5: External tuberosity of the humerus

zxx: M. insfraspinatus

vx: M biceps brachii

6: Deltoid tuberosity of the humerus

g: Anterior portion of the M. pectolaris major

39: M. brachialis internus

8: Olecranon

h: Posterior portions of the M. pectolaris minor

41: M. obliquus abdominis internus

lx: Cartilago scapulae

41: M. obliquus abdominis internus

28:M. quadriceps femoris

20: Depression over the lower part of patella

28x: M. quadriceps femoris

28xx: Trochanter tertius femoris

r: M. semitendinosus

t: Short and long levators of the tail

s: Short and long levators of the tail

31: Posterior part of the sacro-sciatic ligament

p: M. glutaeus medius

16: Tuber coxae

43: M. transversus abdominis

18.R.: 18th rib

m: M. serratus posterior

36: M. longissimus dorsi

37: M. iliocostalis

35: M. spinalis et semispinalis dorsi et cervicis

1x: Cartilago scapulae

x: M. rhomboideus

47: Cervical ligament cord

33: M. complexus

yx: M. longissimus atlantis

y: M. longissimus capitis

*: Border of the atlas

27: Depressor muscle of the auricle

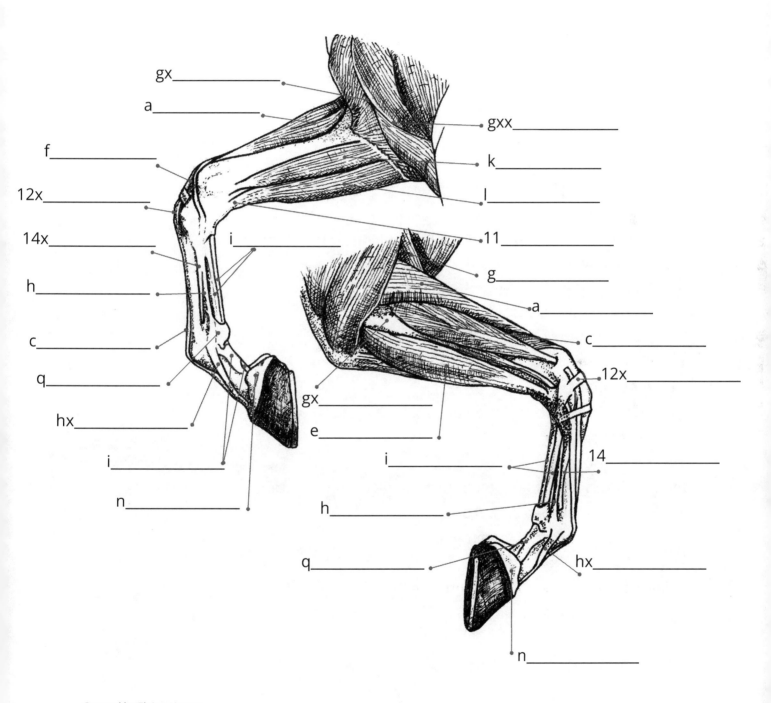

gx_____

a_____

f_____

12x_____

14x_____

h_____

c_____

q_____

hx_____

i_____

n_____

gxx_____

k_____

l_____

11_____

g_____

a_____

c_____

12x_____

gx_____

e_____

i_____

14_____

h_____

q_____

hx_____

n_____

Answers:

gx: End of the M. pectoralis major

a: M extensor carpi radialis

gxx: Same muscle of the left side

f: M. abductor pollicis longus'

12x: Tuberosity of large metacarpal bone

14x: Internal small metacarpal bone

h: M interosseus medius

c: M. extensor digitorum communis

q: Annular ligament

hx: Tendinous band to the tendon of the digitorum communis

i: Flexor tendons

n: Lateral cartilage

k: M. flexor carpi radialis

l: M. extensor carpi ulnaris

11: Os pisiforme

i: Flexor tendons

gx: End of the M. pectoralis major

e: M. extensor carpi ulnaris

n: Lateral cartilage

hx: Tendinous band to the tendon of the digitorum communis

14: Extrenal small metacarpal bone

c: M. extensor digitorum communis

a: M. extensor carpi radialis

g: End of the M. brachialis internus

8_____

gx_____

a_____

gx_____

fx_____

c_____

o_____

e_____

l_____

d_____

K_____

ex_____

11_____

14_____

h_____

i_____

q_____

i_____

n_____

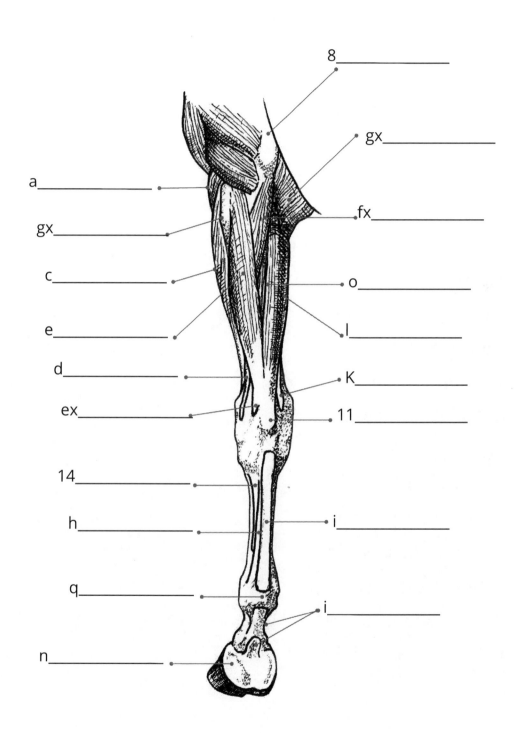

Answers:

a: M. extensor carpi radialis

gx: End of the M. pectoralis major

c: M. extensor digitorum communis

e: M. extensor carpi ulnaris

d: M. extensor digiti minimi

ex: M. extensor carpi ulnaris

14: External small metacarpal bone

h: M interosseus medius

q: Annular ligament

n: Lateral cartilage

i: Flexor tendons

11: Os pisiforme

k: M. flexor carpi radialis

l: M extensor carpi ulnaris

o: M. flexor digitorium profundus

fx: Ulnar head of the deep flexor of the digit

g: End of the end M. brachialis internus

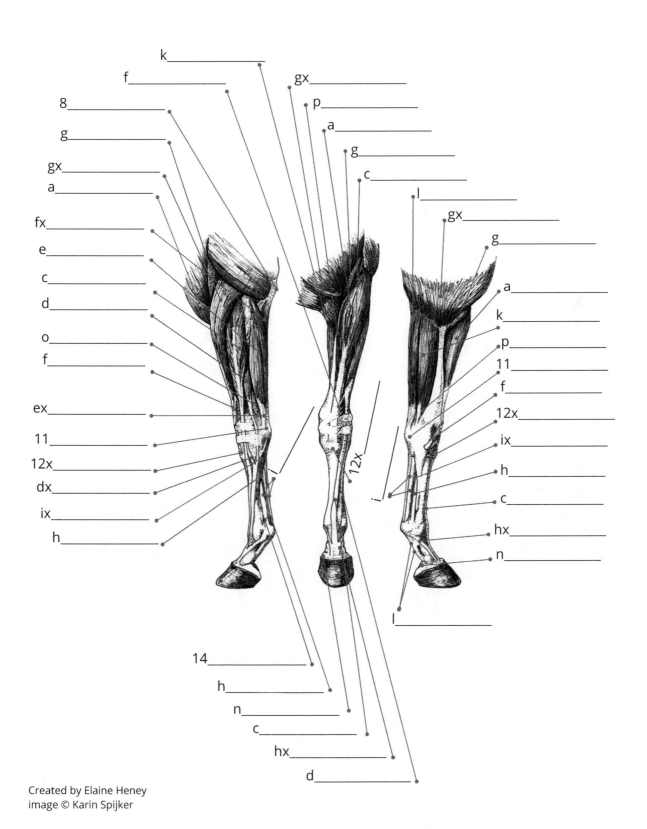

k_____

f_____

gx_____

8_____

p_____

g_____

a_____

gx_____

g_____

a_____

gx_____

c_____

a_____

fx_____

l_____

e_____

gx_____

c_____

g_____

d_____

a_____

o_____

k_____

f_____

p_____

11_____

ex_____

f_____

11_____

12x_____

12x_____

ix_____

dx_____

h_____

ix_____

c_____

h_____

hx_____

i

n_____

12x

i

l_____

14_____

h_____

n_____

c_____

hx_____

d_____

Created by Elaine Heney
image © Karin Spijker

Answers:

8: Olecranon

g: End of the M. brachialis internus

gx: End of the M. pectoralis

a: M. extensor carpi radialis

fx: Ulnar head of the deep flexor of the digit

e: M. extensor carpi ulanaris

c: M. extensor digitorum communis

d: M. extensor digitii minimi

o: M. flexor digitorum profundus

f: M. abductor pollicis longus

ex: M. extensor carpi ulnaris

11: Os pisiforme

12x: Tubersosity of large metacarpal bone

dx: M. extensor digiti minimi

ix: Check ligament

h: M. interosseus medius

14: External small metacarpal bone

h: M. interosseus medius

n: Lateral cartilage

c: M. extensor digitorum communis

hx: Tendinous band to the tendon of the digitorum communis

i: Flexor tendons

k: M. flexor carpi radialis

p: Great subcutaneous vein

a: M. extensor carpi radialis

l: M. extensor carpi ulnaris

ox_____

20_____

q_____

qx_____

qxx_____

r_____

21x_____

36_____

b_____

d_____

21xx_____

i_____

bx_____

dx_____

g_____

ex_____

25xx_____

h_____

l_____

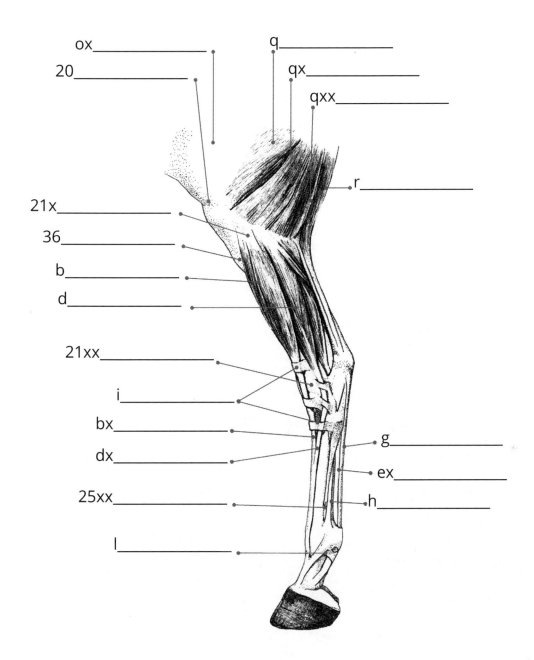

Answers:

ox: Fascia covering the M. quadriceps femoris

20: Patella

21x: External condyle of tibia

36: Crista tibia

b: M. extensor digitorum longus

d: M. extensor digitorum pedis lateralis

21xx: External malleolus of tibia

i: Annular ligaments

bx: M. extensor digitorum longus

dx: M. extensor digitorum pedis lateralis

25xx: Nodular enlarged end of inner small metatarsal bone

l: Tendinous band from the interosseus medius to the common extensor tendon

h: M. interosseus medius

ex: Fusion of tendon and flexor hallucis longus

g: Superficial flexor tendon

r: End of the M. semitendinosus

qxx: End of the M. biceps femoris

qx: End of the M. biceps femoris

q: End of the M. biceps femoris

y_____

x_____   q_____

                         qx_____

20_____

                         21x_____

36_____

a_____   d_____

                         axx_____

21xx_____   i_____

a_____   21xx_____

ax_____   ix_____

b_____   ixx_____

                         dx_____

l_____

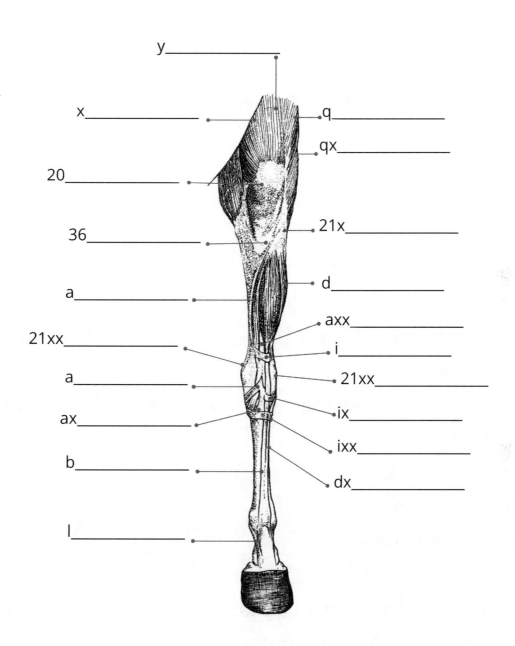

Answers:

y: End of the M. quadriceps femoris

x: End of the M. sartorius

20: Patella

36: Crista tibiae

a: M. tibialis anterior

21xx: External malleoulusof tibia

a: M. tibialis anterior

ax: Inner branch of M. tibialis anterior

b: M. extensor digitorum longus

l: Tendinous band from the interosseus medius to the common extensor tendon

dx: M. extensor digitorum pedis lateralis

i: Annular ligaments

ix: Annular ligaments

21x: Tibia

d: M. extensor digitorum pedis lateralis

qx: End of the M. biceps femoris

q:End of the M. biceps femoris

Answers:

x_____

y_____

20_____

r_____

rx_____

f_____

o_____

fx_____

exx_____

e_____

g_____

21xx_____

m_____

g_____

ex_____

36_____

m_____

b_____

a_____

axx_____

i_____

ax_____

ixx_____

bx_____

h_____

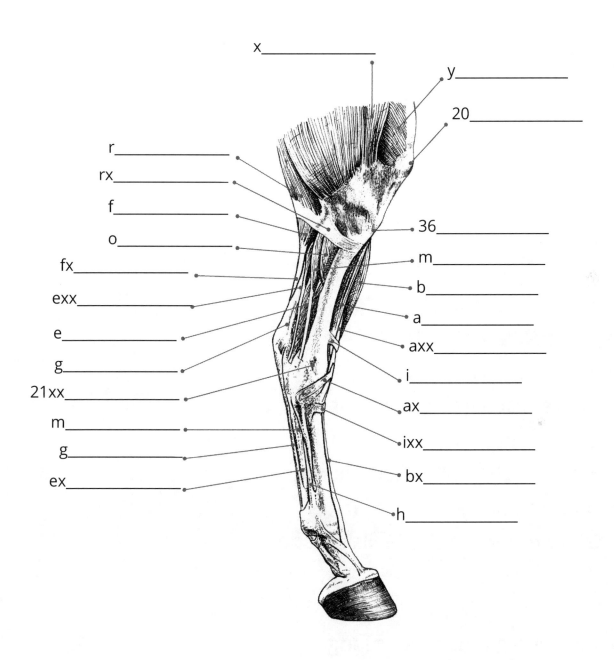

x: End of the M. sartorius

y: End of the M. quadriceps femoris

rx: Tendon of M. semitendinosus

f: Mm. gastrocnemii

o: M. popliteus

fx: Tendo achillis

ex: Fusion of tendon and M. flexor hallucis longus

e: M. flexor hallucis longus

g: Superficial flexor tendon

21xx: External malleolus of tibia

m: M. flexor digitorum pedis longus

g: Superficial flesor tendon

h: M. interosseus medius

bx: M. extensor digitorum longus

ixx: Annular ligaments

ax: Inner branch of M. tibialis anterior

i: Annular ligaments

axx: Outer branch of M. tibialis anterior

a: M. tibialis anterior

b: M. extensor digitorum longus

m: M. flexor digitorum pedis longus

36: Crista tibiae

20: Patella

exx: M. tibalis posterior

r: End of the M. semitendinosus

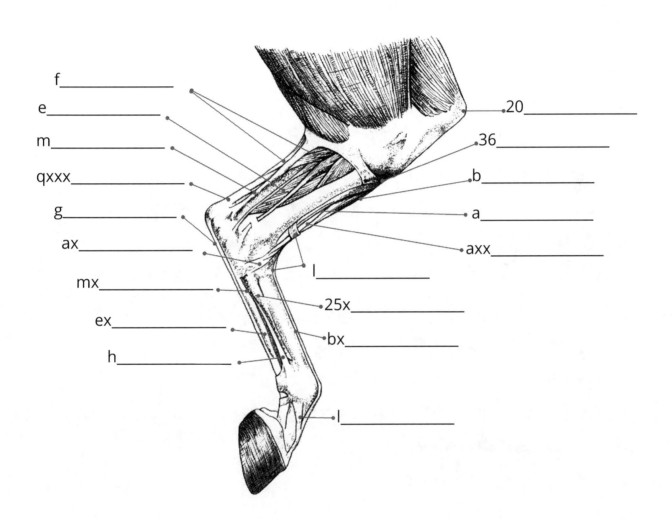

f_____

e_____

m_____

qxxx_____

g_____

ax_____

mx_____

ex_____

h_____

20_____

36_____

b_____

a_____

axx_____

l_____

25x_____

bx_____

l_____

Answers:

f: Mm. gastrocnemii

e: M. flexor hallucis longus

m: M. flexor digitorum pedis longus

qxxx: Tendinous band from M. biceps femoris to fascia of leg

g: Superficial flexor tendon

ax: Inner branch of M. tibialis anterior

mx: Tendon of M. flexor digitorum pedis longus

ex: Fusion of tendon and M. flexor hallucis longus

h: M. interosseus medius

l: Tendinous band from the interosseus medius to the common extensor tendon

bx: M extensor digitorum longus

25x: Inner small metatarsal bone

l: Tendinous band from the interosseus medius to the common extensor tendon

axx: M. peronaeus tertius

a: M. tibialis anterior

b: M extensor digitorum longus

36: Crista tibiae

20: Patella

q_____

qx_____

ox_____

qxx_____

r_____

20_____

21_____

36_____

b_____

i_____

g_____

25x_____

dx_____

h_____

ex_____

l_____

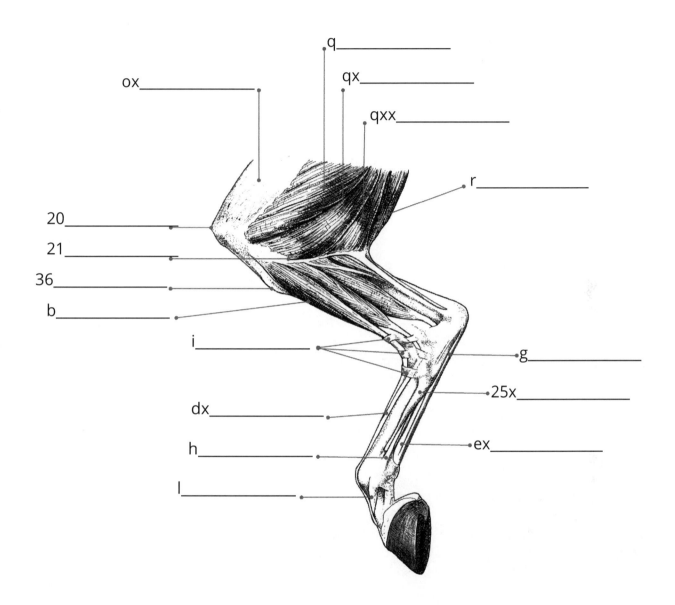

Answers:

ox: Fascia covering the M. quadriceps femoris

20: Patella

21: Tibia

36: Crista tibiae

b: M. extensor digitorum longus

i: Annular ligaments

dx: M extensor digitorum pedis lateralis

h: M. interosseus medius

l: Tendious band from the interosseus medius to the common extensor tendon

ex: Fushion of tendon and M. flexor hallucis longus

25x: Inner small metatarsal bone

g: Superficial flexor tendon

r: End of the M. semitendinosus

qxx: End of the M. biceps femoris

qx: End of the M. biceps femoris

q: End of the M. biceps femoris

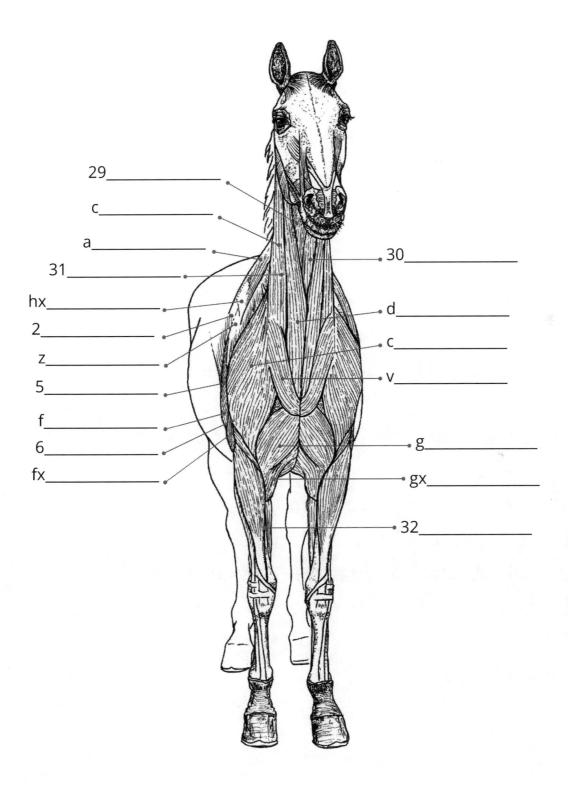

29_____

c_____

a_____

31_____

hx_____

2_____

z_____

5_____

f_____

6_____

fx_____

30_____

d_____

c_____

v_____

g_____

gx_____

32_____

Answers:

29: M. omoyoideus

c: M. cleidomastoideus

a: M. trapezius

31: V. jugularis

hx: Scapular part of M. pectoralis major

2: Spina scapulae

z: M. supraspinatus

5: External tuberosity humerus

f: Caput longum et laterale tricipitis brachii

6: Deltoid tubersosity of humerus (Rotator)

fx: f: Caput longum et laterale tricipitis brachii

32: Cutaneous vein

gx: Sternal part of M. pectoralis major

g: Clavicular part of M. pectoralis major

v: Cervical subcutaneous muscle, (cervical panniculus)

c: M. cleidomastoideus

d: M. sternomandibularis

30: M. sternohyoideus

oxx_____

px_____

t_____

s_____

34_____

19_____

35_____

a_____

h_____

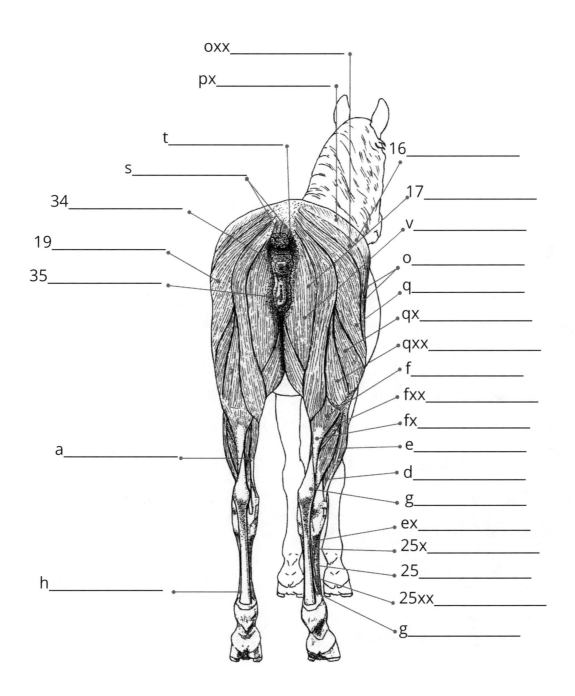

16_____

17_____

v_____

o_____

q_____

qx_____

qxx_____

f_____

fxx_____

fx_____

e_____

d_____

g_____

ex_____

25x_____

25_____

25xx_____

g_____

Answers:

oxx: M. glutaeus maximus

px: Fascia glutaea

t: Muscles of the tail

s: Muscles of the tail

34: Anus

19: Trochanter major of the femur

35: Vulva

a: Inner terminal tendon of M. tibialis anterior

h: M. interosseus medius

g: Superficial flexor tendon

25xx: Capitulum

25: Large cannon bone (3rd metatarsal bone)

25x: External small cannon or splint bone (4th metatarsal bone)

ex: Deep flexor tendon

d: M. extensor digitorum pedis lateralis

e: M. flexor digitorum profundus

fx: Tendo achillis

fxx: M. soleus

f: Terminal part of the united Mm. gastrocnemii

qxx: M. biceps femoris

qx: M. biceps femoris

q: M. biceps femoris

o: M. tensor fasciae latae

v: M semimembranosus

17: tuber ischii

16: Tuber coxae

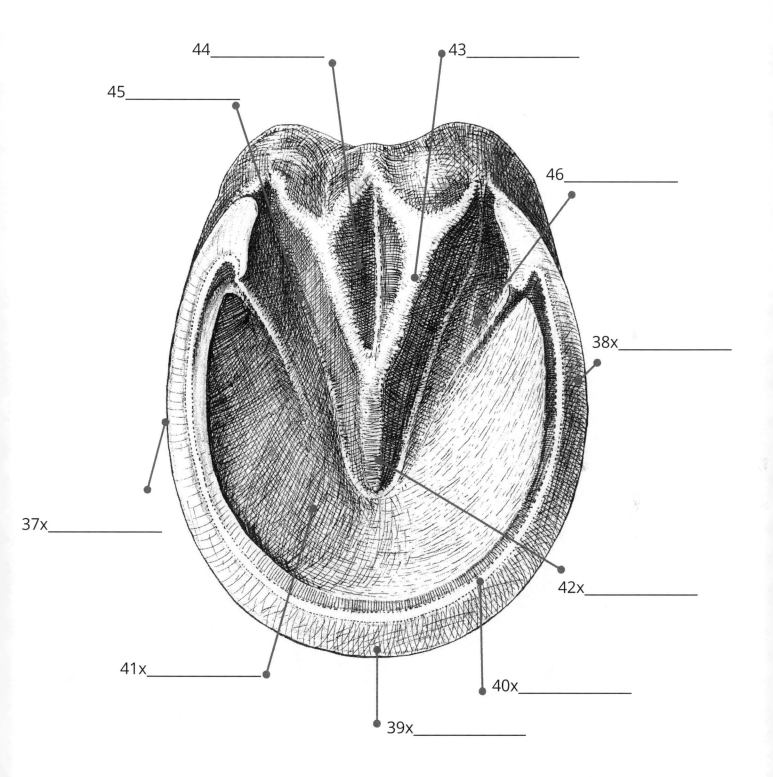

44_____

43_____

45_____

46_____

38x_____

37x_____

42x_____

41x_____

40x_____

39x_____

Created by Elaine Heney
image © Karin Spijker

43: Branch of frog, right fore hoof

44: Median furrow of frog, right fore hoof

45: Lateral furrow of frog, right fore hoof

37x: Inner edge of the lower surface of the sole, right fore hoof

41x: Sole, right fore hoof

39x: Bearing edge, right fore hoof , unshod

40x: So-called white line, right fore hoof

42x: Apex of frog, right fore hoof

38x: Outer edge of the lower surface of the sole, right fore hoof

46: Bar, right fore hoof

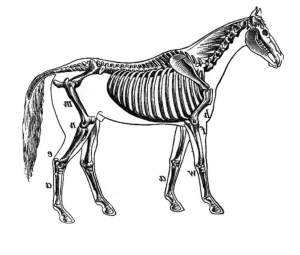

Congratulations

You completed the Horse Anatomy coloring book!

As an independent author, book reviews are a valuable way for you to help me share this book with the world. If you enjoyed this book, I would be hugely grateful if you could share your review & a picture of this book online.
Many thanks, Elaine Heney.

Horse Riding Apps

www.horsestridesapp.com
www.rideableapp.com
www.dressagehero.com
www.poleworkapp.com

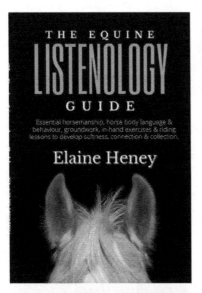
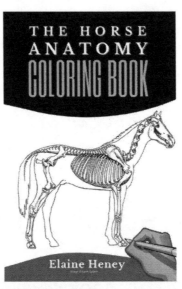
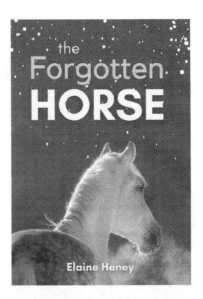
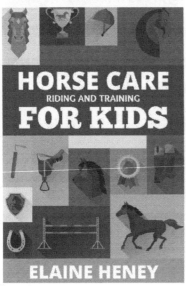
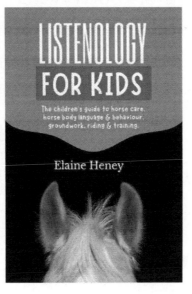
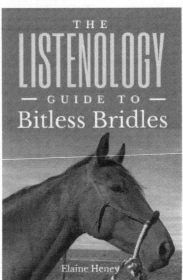

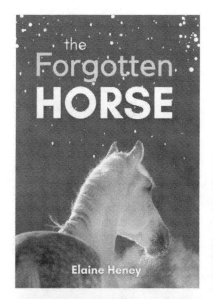
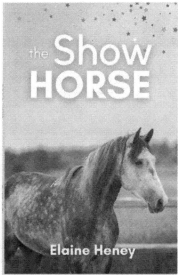
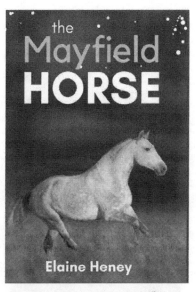
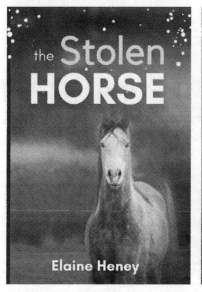
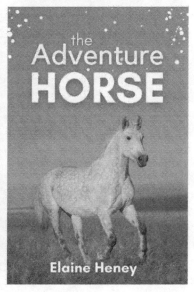
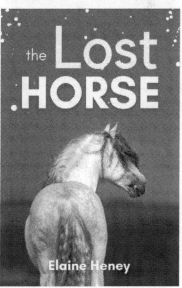